About the Authors

Patricia Coen, co-author of *Beautiful Braids* and *The All-In-One Guide to Natural Foods*, has been a contributing writer/editor for nearly a dozen other books including *Computer Space*, *Pasta & Cheese: The Cookbook*, and *Clothes Care*.

James Wagenvoord is a noted author and photographer whose one-man photography shows have been featured in New York and Boston galleries.

Joe Maxwell is a hairstylist whose client list has included Elizabeth Taylor, Barbra Streisand and Ginger Rogers.

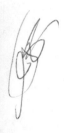

BEAUTIFUL BRAIDS

*The Step-by-Step Guide to Perfect Plaiting For
Every Occasion and All Ages*

by
Patricia Coen
&
Joe Maxwell
&
James Wagenvoord

CENTURY
LONDON SYDNEY AUCKLAND JOHANNESBURG

First published in Great Britain in 1988 by
Century Hutchinson Ltd
Brookmount House, 65-65 Chandos Place, Covent Garden, London
WC2N 4NW

Century Hutchinson Australia (Pty) Ltd
20 Alfred Street, Milsons Point, Sydney, NSW 2061, Australia

Century Hutchinson New Zealand Ltd
PO Box 40-086, 32-34 View Road, Glenfield, Auckland 10, New Zealand

Century Hutchinson South Africa (Pty) Ltd
PO Box 337, Bergvlei 2012, South Africa

Reprinted 1989

Front cover photograph supplied by
Hebe Hair Salon, 38 William IV Street, London WC2

Set in Bembo

Photoset by Deltatype Ltd, Ellesmere Port
Printed and bound in Great Britain by
Courier International Ltd, Tiptree, Essex

British Library Cataloguing in Publication Data

Coen, Patricia
    Beautiful braids: the step-by-step guide to
    perfect plaiting styles for every occasion
    and all ages.
    I. Title   II. Maxwell, Joe
    391'.5

ISBN 0-7126-2399-X

Acknowledgments

Linda Biagi, Nisha Biagi, Pat England, Nell Hanson, Karen Kaufman, Terry Coen, Zandy Hartig, Jennifer Hartig, Kumi Tucker, Linda Raglan Cunningham, Maureen Kelly, Linda Hodgson, Lindsay Hodgson, James and Carole Hunt, Lisa Spadaro, Morgan Thomas, Dianne Hughes, Wendy McCurdy, Anita Wagenvoord, Catherine Greenman, Tommy Alessi, Berkey K&L, Marion Zimmer, Laura Woodworth, Lynn Kenny, Karina Kindler.

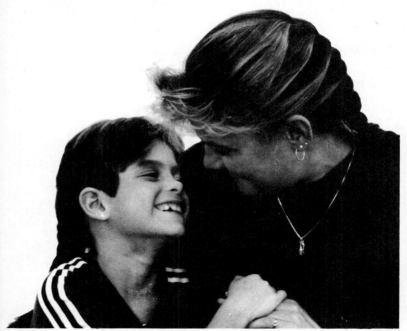

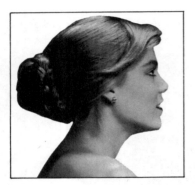

Cameo

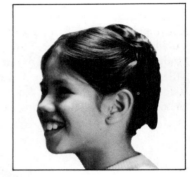

Tiara

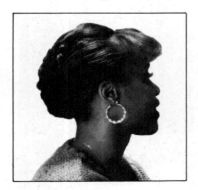

Evensong

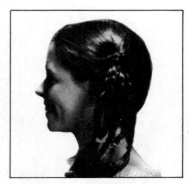

Simplified Cornrows

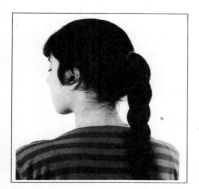

English Braid

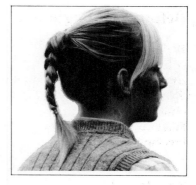

Dutch Braid

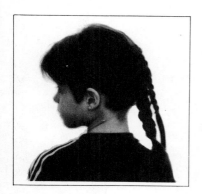

Double English Braid

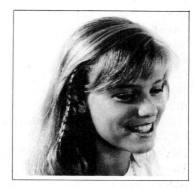

Single French
Accent Braid

Contents

Contents

Before You Begin . . .

Braids are popular, and they deserve to be. They look good on women of all ages, shapes and sizes. And they're surprisingly versatile. Using easy braiding techniques, you can create literally dozens of elegant hairstyles and looks.

Braids aren't just for long hair. If your hair is chin-length or even slightly shorter, you can use delicate English, Dutch or French braids as accents. If your hair is shoulder-length or longer, you can create any of the braided looks featured in **Beautiful Braids**.

Braids are practical. A properly fashioned braid will stay neatly in place from morning until night, leaving you free to pursue any activity you choose without reaching for a comb. An English braid worn to keep your hair neat during an afternoon tennis match can easily be coiled into a chignon for evening. If your hair is in the process of growing out, leaving you with uneven wisps around your face, you can braid it to keep it swept back. In hot weather, you can fashion any one of a number of braids and pin it up, so your hair will stay off your face and neck.

Although the braided look is as new as today, braids have a long history. In Africa, elaborate braided styles (the forerunners of modern corn rows) were sculpted on to the head and decorated with beads and precious stones to mark rites of passage for both men and women.

In medieval Europe, long, flowing hair was prized as a virgin's attribute. Then, as now, young women devoted hours to pampering their hair with herbs and medications, using combs carved from wood and ivory. Their braids were arranged in a variety of styles—hanging loose down the back, coiled atop the head or curled into braided earmuffs.

Before You Begin . . .

Braids retained their popularity in Europe throughout the Renaissance, the styles changing slightly with the times. Braids were wrapped around the head either horizontally or vertically, and small, delicate braids were woven throughout the hair as decoration.

During the Victorian era, braids were arranged to complement that period's demure clothing styles. Braided hair was looped down beside the cheeks and back up over the ears, or coiled in large loops at the back of the head.

Any historical style can be adopted by modern women, along with any of the dozens of braid variations. The beauty of braids is their versatility and simplicity. Once you've mastered a few very basic steps, you can fashion **any** kind of braid, and even begin to create your own styles. Braids are flattering to everyone, and they can be anything you want them to be—innocent, sophisticated, and everything in between.

Braiding Tips

The results of braiding appear intricate, but the techniques are simple. Braiding is a skill that you can easily learn with just a little practice and patience. A few basic techniques, once mastered, will enable you to create both simple and elaborate braids. During your first few attempts at braiding, you'll begin to learn the rhythms of the techniques. Braiding is just the repetition of a simple weaving pattern, and this pattern will soon become natural and comfortable for you.

Visualization is the key to braiding. Before you attempt even one plait, look at the step-by-step instructions beginning on page 17. Imagine yourself carrying out each step on your own hair. Braid your hair at first only in your imagination. Visualization is important even after you begin to braid; as you work, give your complete attention to each step, picturing exactly what the step should look like as you do it and when it's completed. This will keep you from becoming confused as you work.

Before You Begin . . .

Don't watch yourself in a mirror as you braid—the reversed image will be misleading. Simply concentrate on what you're doing. Close your eyes to eliminate distractions. When you're finished, check the results in a mirror. Don't be discouraged if there are stray hairs. After you've braided a few times, your touch will become sensitive enough to feel any hairs that are out of place.

Always work with damp hair, or hair that is at least slightly damp. It holds together easily, leaving fewer stray hairs to worry about.

Use a covered rubber band to secure your hair in a ponytail when you try your first braids. Other accessories you'll find useful are clips or barrettes to hold sections of hair out of your way while you're braiding others, and bobby pins or hairpins to anchor styles like the Chignon and the Invisible French braid.

Relax. Many people unconsciously tense their shoulder muscles as they hold their hands up to braid because the position seems unfamiliar. You'll be more comfortable if you avoid this tendency to tighten up.

Keep even tension on all the strands of hair as you braid.

Don't worry about taking the "right" amount of hair for each plait. While the strands should be of about equal thickness to begin with, they needn't be absolutely uniform for the braid to turn out properly.

Take it easy. If you make a mistake, there's no harm done. It will only take a moment for you to unbraid your hair and begin again.

A Braider's Glossary

Braid—To interlace or entwine; strands of hair that have been interlaced or entwined to form a pattern.

Chignon—Hair gathered and fastened together to give the appearance of a knot or bun. Usually worn at the crown or nape.

Crown—The topmost part of the head. To locate the crown, place the tips of your index fingers above your ears and draw the fingers upward. The point at which they meet on the top rear portion of your head is the crown.

Fringe—Hair cut short to fall over the forehead.

Hairline—The line around the face (temple to forehead to temple) where hair begins to grow.

Nape—The back of the neck, at the base of the hairline.

Plait—One complete step in the braiding sequence, i.e., left over centre and right over centre.

Sectioning—Dividing the portion of hair you plan to work with from the rest of the hair.

Strands—The sections of hair that are twined together to form a braid. The hair is divided into three strands to fashion a typical braid.

Texture—The characteristic surface of the hair. Fine hair has a different texture than thick hair, and different textures may be suited to different kinds of braids.

Establishing a Hair-Care Routine

The woven, coiled patterns you create in braiding are enormously enhanced by glossy, manageable hair. Getting your hair in top condition is simple, requiring only a few minutes each day and some common sense. Once you've established a sensible hair-care routine, your braids will always be beautiful.

Everyone's hair is one of three types—dry, normal, or oily—and each type requires slightly different care. For example, daily shampooing may be too drying for hair that tends to be dry, but it won't harm normal hair, and it may be essential to keep oily hair looking clean. Nearly every name-brand shampoo and conditioner is available in three formulas, one for each hair type.

Shampoos & Conditioners

Generally, how often you shampoo depends on your hair type,

Before You Begin . . .

environment, and activities. Regardless of hair type, you should always shampoo after exposing your hair to chlorinated pool water or salt water, or when you've increased the amount of perspiration present on your scalp by strenuous exercise or by spending time in the sun.

The instructions on most shampoos tell you to lather and rinse your hair twice. Ignore them. One lathering should be enough to clean your hair without stripping its essential natural oils or drying your scalp.

Normal hair can be shampooed daily, although this isn't necessary unless you live in a large city, where dirt and pollution tend to deposit on hair. Use any shampoo formulated for normal hair, with or without a conditioning agent. You may want to use a separate conditioner on normal hair every third or fourth shampoo to keep it at its best.

Oily hair should be shampooed every day, especially in urban areas or humid climates. Use shampoos formulated for oily hair and avoid those that contain conditioning agents, which tend to leave a slightly greasy residue in oily hair.

Dry hair should be washed as infrequently as possible because the detergents and soaps present in all shampoos strip hair of its essential natural oils. Select a shampoo formulated for dry hair, preferably one with a conditioning agent. Special conditioning is necessary to keep dry, flyaway hair under control.

Conditioners make hair shinier, more manageable, and tangle free. Nearly all conditioners contain some form of protein that coats hair shafts to make them thicker and give the hair body. This coating action is more valuable for some hair types than others.

Normal hair and **dry hair** benefit from conditioning. A conditioner will "build up" hair, particularly if it is thin or limp. Dry hair, which tends to be unruly and difficult to manage after shampooing, can be calmed and made shinier by a conditioner.

Oily hair usually gains no benefits from conditioners. Coating the shafts of oily hair sometimes makes it oilier, although some

Before You Begin . . .

conditioners are formulated especially for oily hair to reduce this tendency.

There are dozens of brands of conditioners. If you use any one brand for more than a month, however, your hair can become immune to its formula, reducing its effectiveness. Each brand combines necessary conditioning agents in different quantities and formulations, and you can avoid building up an immunity to a specific conditioner simply by switching brands. It's best to find three brands that work well for you and use one for a month, then switch to another for the second month and to another for the third. In the fourth month, you can safely return to the first brand.

Grooming & Styling

Treat wet hair gently. Wet hair is weak and can be easily stretched or snapped, resulting in split ends and flyaway hair. Always use a large wide-toothed comb to groom wet hair, as a brush is likely to catch in the hair and snap it.

Although blow dryers are convenient for quick drying, they should be used sparingly. Don't use a blow dryer every day—this will simply dry out your hair too much, even if it's oily. Two or three times a week should be the maximum. To expose your hair to as little potentially damaging heat as possible, let it dry naturally for at least a few minutes before using a blow dryer.

Hair needs to be brushed, but not for the traditional one hundred strokes each day. Twenty-five strokes are sufficient to smooth it and distribute natural oils—any more than that, and you run the risk of damaging the roots.

Finger & Hand Positions

The methods you will use to braid your hair are the same techniques used to braid or weave yarn, rope or any other material. Braiding is

Before You Begin . . .

simply taking three sections of hair and crossing the outside sections over and into the centre. As you work, the sections of hair are interwoven to create plaits.

A braid is composed of a series of simple "cross-take-tighten-return" sequences, using motions that flow naturally from and into one another. A complete sequence takes only a few seconds.

There is no one "right" way to braid. Every braider develops individual finger and hand positions that are comfortable and successful for her. Illustrated here are basic positions that act as a starting place or reference point.

The illustrations show the beginning of an English braid, with your hands in position at the back of your head. Obviously, to fashion a braid on the side of your head, your arms and hands will be placed somewhat differently; that's an adaptation you can easily make yourself after you're comfortable with the fundamentals. Remember, ultimately it's what happens to the hair—not the exact finger and hand positions—that's important.

Before You Begin . . .

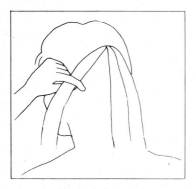

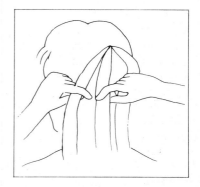

1 Take the left strand in your hand, between your thumb and first finger. The three fingers behind it are free.

2 Hold the centre strand between your right thumb and first finger and the right strand with your last two fingers.

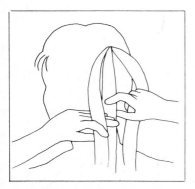

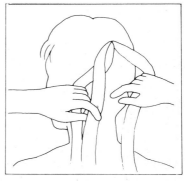

3 **CROSS**. Cross the left strand over the centre strand, holding it slightly above the centre strand.

4 **TAKE**. Loop the free fingers of your left hand over the centre strand and take it from your right hand.

Before You Begin . . .

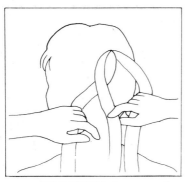

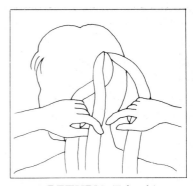

5 **TIGHTEN**. Use your free right thumb and first finger to take the centre strand and pull it gently, ensuring that the first half-plait is taut.

6 **RETURN**. Take this new centre strand back between the thumb and first finger of your left hand. You're now holding two strands in your left hand and one in your right.

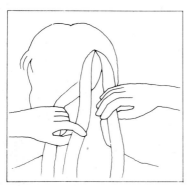

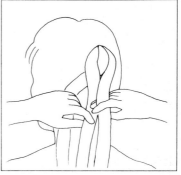

7 Move that strand so that you're holding it between your right thumb and first finger (if you need to let go of the strand to position it properly, go ahead).

8 **CROSS**. Cross the right strand over the centre strand, holding it slightly above the centre strand.

Now, repeat the "cross-take-tighten-return" sequence, beginning with your right hand.

Before You Begin . . .

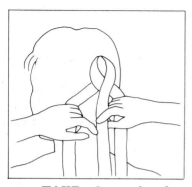

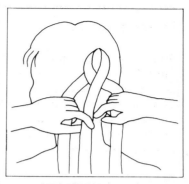

9 **TAKE**. Loop the free fingers of your right hand over the centre strand and take it from your left hand.

10 **TIGHTEN**. Use your free left thumb and first finger to take the strand and pull it gently.

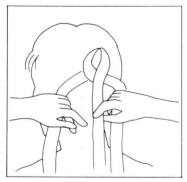

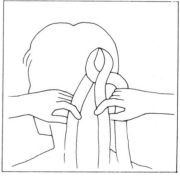

11 **RETURN**. Take this new centre strand back between the thumb and first finger of your right hand. You now have two strands in your right hand and one in your left, held by the last two fingers.

12 Move that strand so that you're holding it between your left thumb and first finger.

Your hands have returned to their starting positions, except that you now have one plait, the beginning of a braid.

Before You Begin . . .

Freeing a Hand

While you're braiding, you'll occasionally need a free hand to smooth the strands you're working with or to make sure a plait feels taut. It's not difficult to hold all three strands in one hand, separated by your fingers. Remember that as you braid, you'll always have two strands in one hand and one in the other. The hand holding a single strand is the one that you should free. These illustrations show a braider freeing one hand.

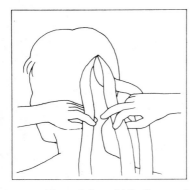

1 Extend the middle finger of the hand holding two strands.

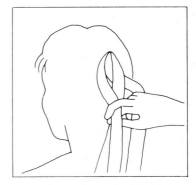

2 Cross the single strand over the centre. Curl the middle finger around it, holding it between and slightly above the other two strands.

Before You Begin . . .

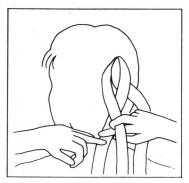

3 To resume braiding, use the last two fingers of your free hand to take the centre strand from between the thumb and first finger of your other hand.

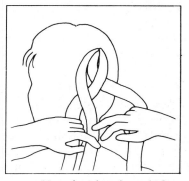

4 Use the thumb and first finger of the hand that you freed to remove the strand held by the middle finger. This makes it the new centre strand.

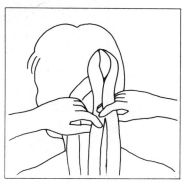

5 You've completed half a plait. Move the single strand from between the last two fingers to between the thumb and first finger and continue braiding.

The Braids

Every braid, from the simplest to the most complex, is created from the English, Dutch or French braid. Once you've mastered these easy-to-learn techniques, even the most elaborate braid will seem simple. Each technique shown is slightly more advanced (not more difficult) than the one before it, and each braid can stand alone as an attractive style or be used in combination with others. You can use these instructions to braid your own hair or a friend's.

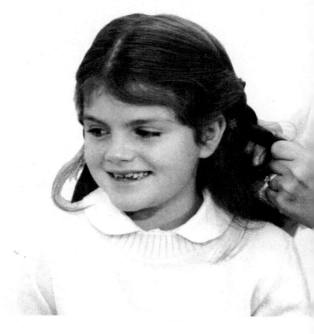

The Braids

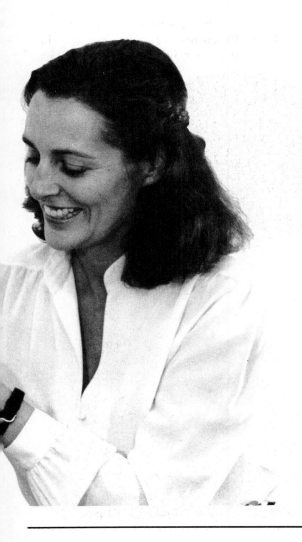

English Braid

English Braid

The simplest braid is the English braid—the same one that was begun in the **Finger & Hand Positions** section on page 17. This versatile three-strand braid is an element of many different styles.

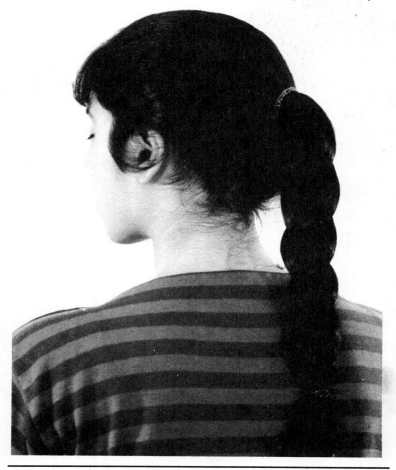

English Braid

Once you're comfortable with the English braid, fashioning any other braid will be easy.

In your first attempts at the English braid, gather your hair into a ponytail and secure it with a covered rubber band. This will help you keep the base of the braid tightly against your scalp. You'll have to

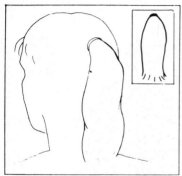

1 Brush your hair back into a ponytail with its base slightly below your crown.

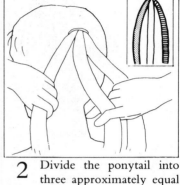

2 Divide the ponytail into three approximately equal strands and position your fingers to begin braiding.

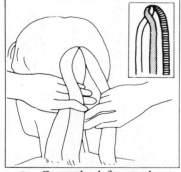

3 Cross the left strand over the centre taking the centre strand to the left, so that the two strands trade places.

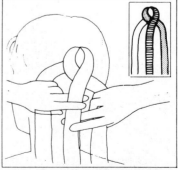

4 Cross the right strand over the centre, taking the centre strand to the right, so that these two strands trade places.

English Braid

leave the band on after the braid is completed, but you can camouflage it by using a colour that's close to your hair colour. Or you can coil the braid into a chignon (see page 28) to hide it. With practice, you'll be able to begin a braid neatly without the rubber

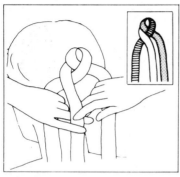

5 Cross the left strand over the centre taking the centre strand to the left.

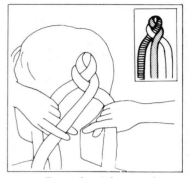

6 Cross the right strand over the centre, taking the centre strand to the right.

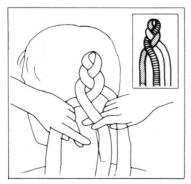

7 Cross the left strand over the centre, taking the centre strand to the left.

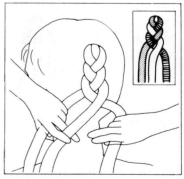

8 Cross the right strand over the centre, taking the centre strand to the right.

band, simply keeping the first plait very tight against the scalp to act as a foundation.

As you become more comfortable with braiding, you can modify the techniques shown to find the method that suits you best.

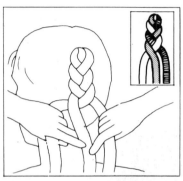

9 Cross the left strand over the centre, taking the centre strand to the left.

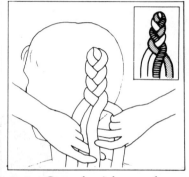

10 Cross the right strand over the centre, taking the centre strand to the right.

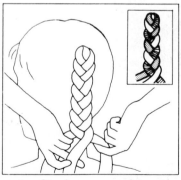

11 Continue crossing the strands alternately over the centre, until the braid is as long as you want it.

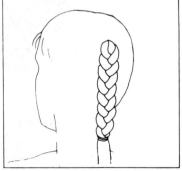

12 Fasten the end with a covered rubber band.

English Braid with Chignon

English Braid with Chignon

In just a few steps, you can turn the basic English braid into an elegant hairstyle. If you've used a covered rubber band to anchor the

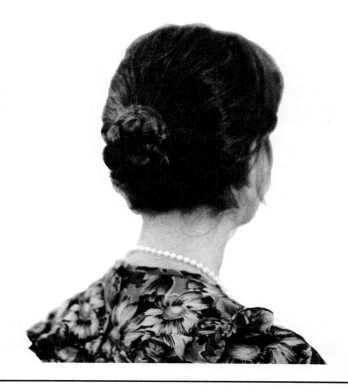

English Braid with Chignon

base of your English braid, creating a chignon will conceal it. Follow the instructions for the English braid on page 24 and then carry out the following steps.

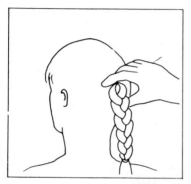

1 Place your index finger against your head, touching the base of the braid.

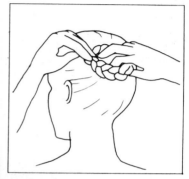

2 Coil the braid around the finger, encircling the base of the braid.

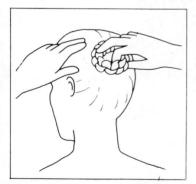

3 Tuck the end of the braid underneath the coil of hair that you've created.

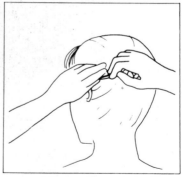

4 Cup the coiled braid in your hand and use hairpins to secure it tightly to your scalp.

Dutch Braid

Dutch Braid

The Dutch braid is essentially a backward English braid. The strands are crossed under, rather than over, the centre, so the first plait isn't fitted as closely against the scalp as it is in English braiding. The finished braid appears slightly flat and loose because the plaits are really upside down.

As with the English braid, begin your first few attempts at the Dutch braid with a ponytail anchored by a covered rubber band.

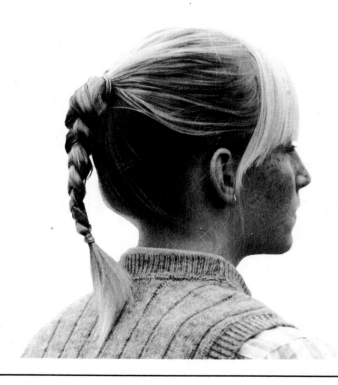

Dutch Braid

You'll be able to give your full attention to mastering the art of crossing the strands underneath one another. You can use the finger and hand positions illustrated on page 17 or devise your own. Once

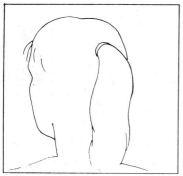

1 Brush your hair back into a ponytail with its base slightly below your crown.

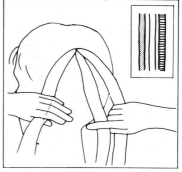

2 Divide the ponytail into three approximately equal strands and position your fingers to begin braiding.

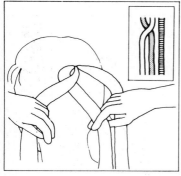

3 Cross the left strand under the centre, taking the centre strand to the left, so that the two strands trade places.

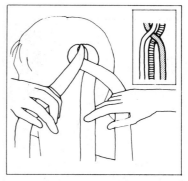

4 Cross the right strand under the centre taking the centre strand to the right, so that these two strands trade places.

Dutch Braid

you're comfortable with the braid itself, beginning it neatly won't be a problem.

Attractive on its own, the Dutch braid is also an important

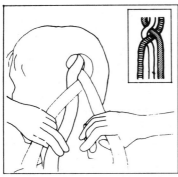

5 Cross the left strand under the centre, taking the centre strand to the left.

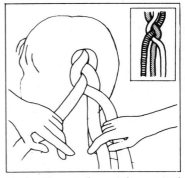

6 Cross the right strand under the centre, taking the centre strand to the right.

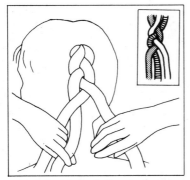

7 Cross the left strand under the centre taking the centre strand to the left.

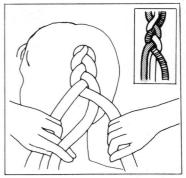

8 Cross the right strand under the centre, taking the centre strand to the right.

Dutch Braid

element of several more elaborate braid styles, including the elegant Underbraid on page 64. It offers almost endless variations and possibilities for experimentation.

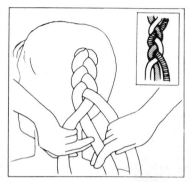

9 Cross the left strand under the centre, taking the centre strand to the left.

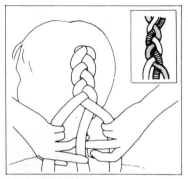

10 Cross the right strand under the centre, taking the centre strand to the right.

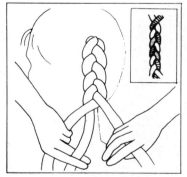

11 Continue crossing the strands alternately under the centre until the braid is as long as you want it.

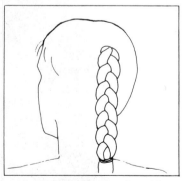

12 Fasten the end with a covered rubber band.

French Braid

French Braid

The French braid, one of the best-known braids, is admired for its elegant, sophisticated look. Its complex appearance is deceiving; it is, in fact, extremely easy to create. It is essentially an English braid with an additional step.

The French braid begins with a thin ponytail skimmed from the top layer of your hair. As you braid, you'll gather additional hair and

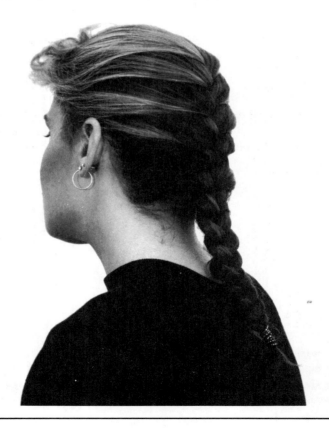

French Braid

add it to the strands. These additions result in gracefully draped hair on either side of the braid. The appearance of the drape varies with the amount of hair you add and the tension you keep on each strand.

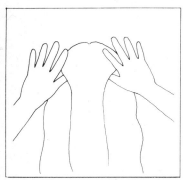

1 Place your thumbs above and behind your ears. Draw your thumbs slightly back and upward, gathering hair that meets at your crown in a ponytail.

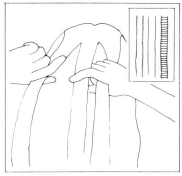

2 Divide the ponytail into three approximately equal sections and position your fingers to begin braiding.

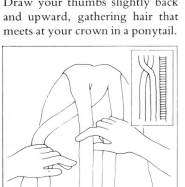

3 Cross the left strand over the centre, taking the centre strand to the left, so that the two strands trade places.

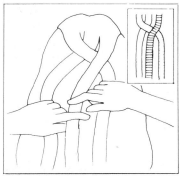

4 Cross the right strand over the centre, taking the centre strand to the right, so that these two strands trade places.

French Braid

Experiment and see what works best for you.

Visualization is essential to all braiding, but especially to French braiding. Because you're dealing with more than three strands for

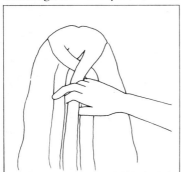

5 Hold the plait in your right hand, separating the three loose strands below it with your fingers.

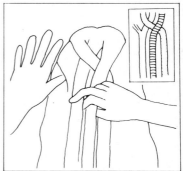

6 Place your left thumb above and behind your left ear. Draw a strand half as thick as one of the original strands toward the ponytail.

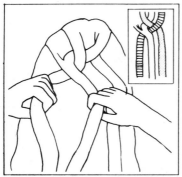

7 Add the newly gathered hair to the left strand. Cross the increased left strand over the centre, taking the centre strand to the left.

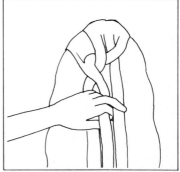

8 Hold the plait in your left hand, separating the three loose strands below it with your fingers.

French Braid

the first time, the gathering step initially requires your full attention. Read through the instructions once and then perform each step on your own hair, concentrating on how it should look.

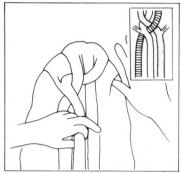

9 Use your right thumb to draw a strand of hair about half as thick as one of the original strands up towards the ponytail.

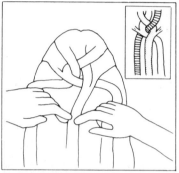

10 Add the newly gathered hair to the right strand. Cross the increased right strand over the centre, taking the centre strand to the right.

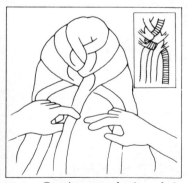

11 Continue gathering hair from the left and right and adding it to the strands just before you cross them over the centre.

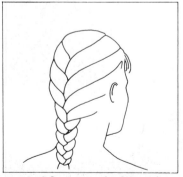

12 After several plaits, there will be no loose hair left to gather. English-braid the remaining strands.

Invisible French Braid

Invisible French Braid

The Invisible French braid is one of the most elegant of all braided looks. Although it's appropriate for everyday, it's also ideal for even the most formal occasion. It begins with a regular French Braid (illustrated on page 34).

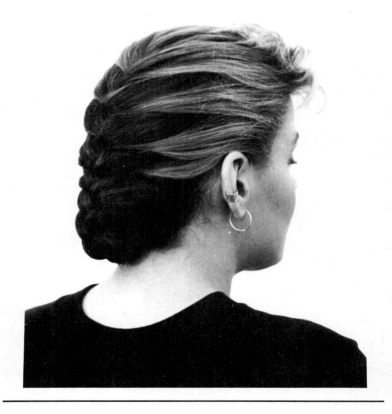

Invisible French Braid

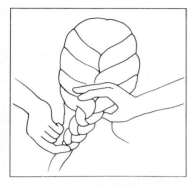

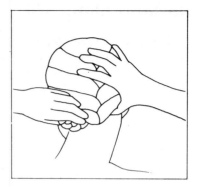

1 Take the hanging, English-braided portion of the standard French braid in your hand.

2 Fold it in toward your neck, tucking it up underneath the French braid, lined up between the gathers.

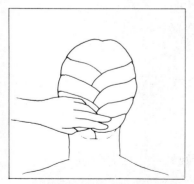

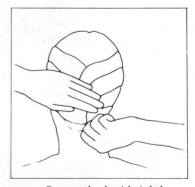

3 The hanging braid is hidden underneath the French braid, against your scalp.

4 Secure the braid tightly to your scalp with hairpins.

Double English Braid

Double English Braid

Even the most basic braids can be used to create unusual styles. Double English braids (you can also use Dutch braids to create this style) are an excellent example of braids' versatility.

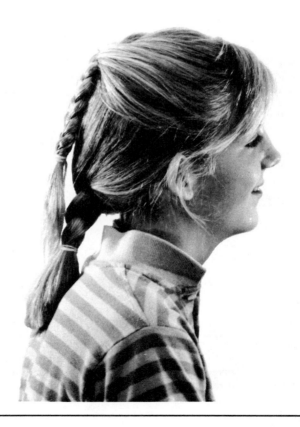

Double English Braid

Double English braids use the basic English braiding technique, yet the final effect is very different from that of an "ordinary" English braid. By stacking two English braids, one on top of the

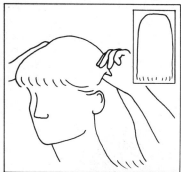

1 Place your thumbs slightly in front of and above your ears, near your temples.

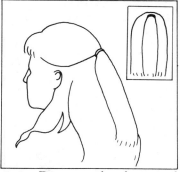

2 Draw your thumbs upward to your crown, gathering the top layer of hair into a thin ponytail with its base at your crown.

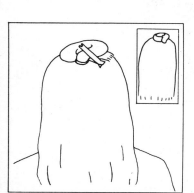

3 You'll work with the loose hair first, so secure the ponytail with a covered rubber band and clip it to the top of your head.

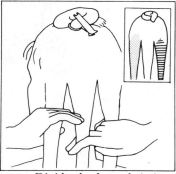

4 Divide the loose hair into three approximately equal strands and position your fingers to begin braiding.

Double English Braid

other, you can create a unique, casual look.

Like most braids, the Double English braid has its practical side. It is ideal for very thick hair that might pull too heavily on the head if

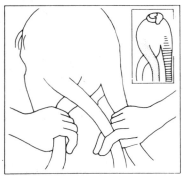

5 Cross the left strand over the centre, taking the centre strand to the left.

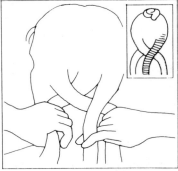

6 Cross the right strand over the centre, taking the centre strand to the right.

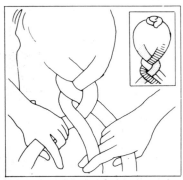

7 Continue crossing the strands alternately over the centre. Fasten the end of the completed braid with a covered rubber band.

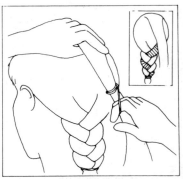

8 Unpin the top ponytail and remove its covered rubber band.

Double English Braid

it's worn in one braid. However, thick or especially long hair is not a necessity for creating successful Double English braids—you need only shoulder-length hair.

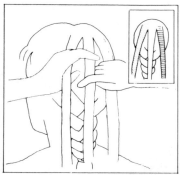

9 Divide the loose hair into three approximately equal strands and position your fingers to begin braiding.

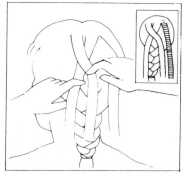

10 Cross the left strand over the centre, taking the centre strand to the left.

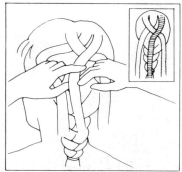

11 Cross the right strand over the centre, taking the centre strand to the right.

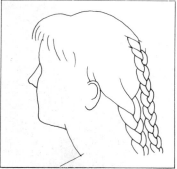

12 Continue crossing the strands alternately over the centre. Fasten the end of the completed braid with a covered rubber band.

Double Dutch Tieback

Double Dutch Tieback

The Double Dutch Tieback is one of the most practical and versatile of all braids. (You can also use English braids to create this style.) Fashionable and attractive, it has the added advantage of keeping all your hair—both braided and loose—pulled neatly back from your face.

Using the basic Dutch braiding technique, you can create a variety of looks by beginning with different sized sections of hair. A very

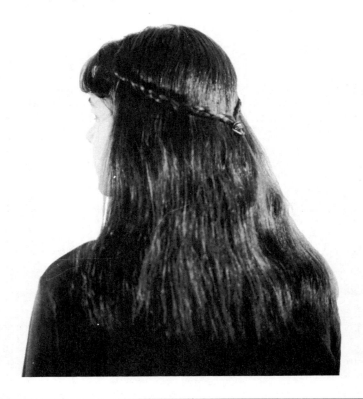

Double Dutch Tieback

thin section will give you tiny braids that ornament your hair; thicker sections will yield more substantial braids.

The Double Dutch Tieback lets you use your imagination. The

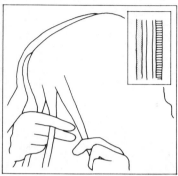

1 Section off a strand of hair approximately ½″ in diameter on one side of your face. Divide it into three approximately equal strands.

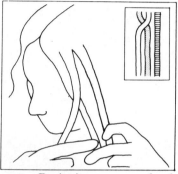

2 Beginning at eye level, cross the right strand under the centre, taking the centre strand to the right. Pull the strands taut.

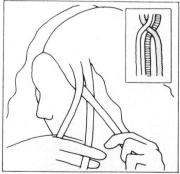

3 Cross the left strand under the centre, taking the centre strand to the left. Make sure the strands are taut.

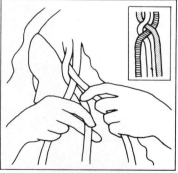

4 Cross the right strand under the centre, taking the centre strand to the right. Make sure the strands are taut.

Double Dutch Tieback

braids can be worn loose; you can fasten them with a covered rubber band or hair clip; you can pin each one back separately or, if your hair is long enough, you can even knot them loosely together.

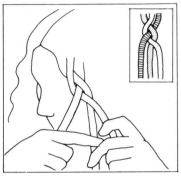

5 Cross the left strand under the centre strand, taking the centre strand to the left. Make sure the strands are taut.

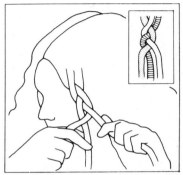

6 Cross the right strand under the centre, taking the centre strand to the right. Make sure the strands are taut.

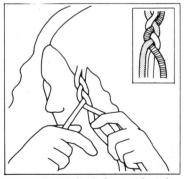

7 Cross the left strand under the centre, taking the centre strand to the left.

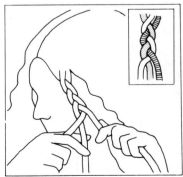

8 Cross the right strand under the centre, taking the centre strand to the right.

Double Dutch Tieback

The Double Dutch Tieback looks its best when you take care to make the plaits smooth and delicate. Begin braiding on either side of your face.

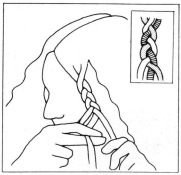

9 Cross the left strand under the centre, taking the centre strand to the left.

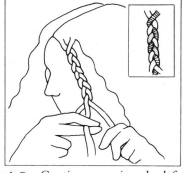

10 Continue crossing the left and then the right strands alternately under the centre until the strands are too short to braid. ▪

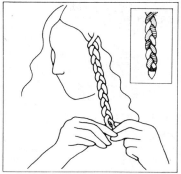

11 Fasten the end with a small covered rubber band. Repeat the steps to fashion another braid on the other side of your face.

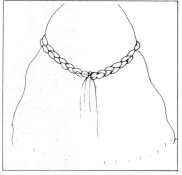

12 You can wear the braids loose, but you'll get a more striking look if you fasten them at the back of your head, sweeping your hair off your face.

Single French Accent Braid

Single French Accent Braid

The Single French Accent braid is especially easy for the beginner, because you can watch what you're doing as you braid—without using a mirror. Popular with teenagers, the Single French Accent braid gives loose hair a "dressed-up" look.

As practical as it is pretty, this accent braid solves the problem of overgrown fringes. Shorter hairs can be woven in with longer ones

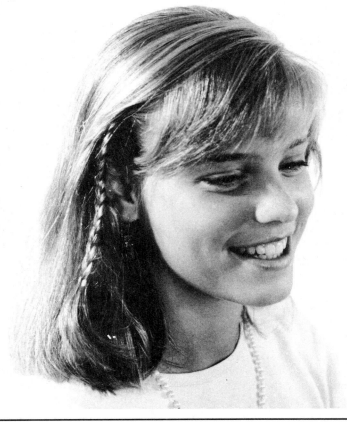

Single French Accent Braid

and held cleanly back from your face.

The Single French Accent braid uses both an English and a modified French braiding technique. You can make the braid as thin

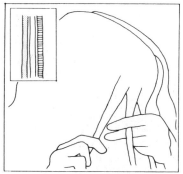

1 Section off a portion of hair about ¼" in diameter right next to your face. Divide the section into three equal strands.

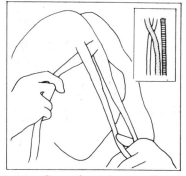

2 Cross the right strand over the centre, taking the centre strand to the right. Pull the strands taut.

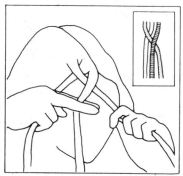

3 Cross the left strand over the centre, taking the centre strand to the left. Make sure the strands are taut.

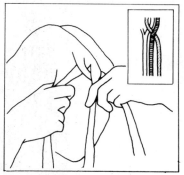

4 Gather a very thin section of hair from the loose hair hanging behind the braid and add it to the right strand.

Single French Accent Braid

or as thick as you like, depending on the amount of hair you begin with. The key to a beautiful accent braid is to pull the strands you're braiding extremely tight to accentuate the braid's delicate quality.

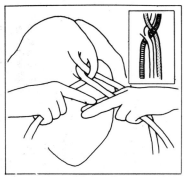

5 Cross the increased right strand over the centre, taking the centre strand to the right.

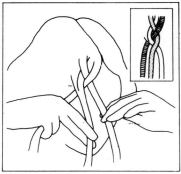

6 Cross the left strand over the centre, taking the centre strand to the left.

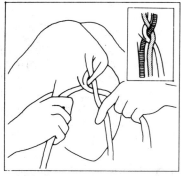

7 Gather another thin section of hair from the loose hair hanging behind the braid.

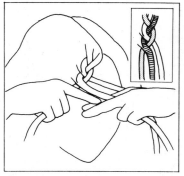

8 Add the newly gathered hair to the right section and cross the increased right strand over the centre.

Single French Accent Braid

You can fashion more than one accent braid and place them anywhere you please. In these illustrations, the braid is being formed on the right-hand side of the face.

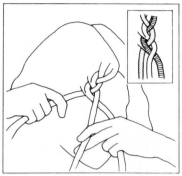

9 Cross the left strand over the centre, taking the centre strand to the left.

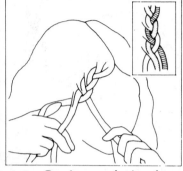

10 Continue gathering loose hair, adding it to the right, and crossing the left and right strands alternately over the centre.

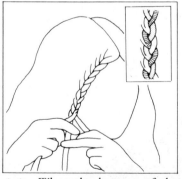

11 When the bottom of the braided hair is about level with your eye, English-braid the loose strands below the French plaits.

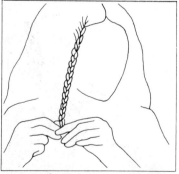

12 Fasten the end of the braid with a covered rubber band. It can be worn loose near the face or pinned back for a more sophisticated look.

Braided Face Frame

Braided Face Frame

The Braided Face Frame combines two braiding techniques, English and French, resulting in a stunning style that's flattering to everyone. It's also ideal for blending uneven wisps near your face—or a fringe that is growing out—in with the rest of your hair, eliminating loose strands.

The key to fashioning a successful Braided Face Frame is starting

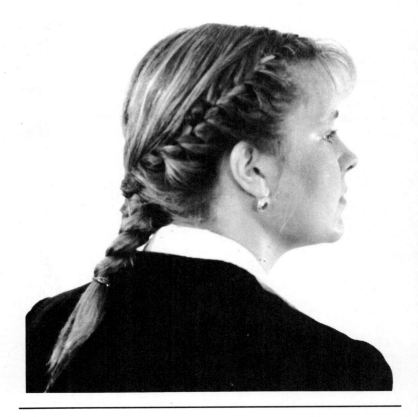

Braided Face Frame

it right. Remember to begin your first plait by crossing the strand nearest your face over the centre to support the braid from underneath and keep it in place.

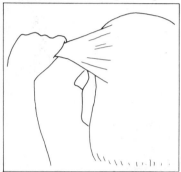

1   Section off a thin portion of hair from your hairline, at your temple. Divide the section into three equal strands.

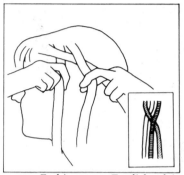

2   Fashion one English plait by crossing the strand closest to your face, and then the one farthest from your face, over the centre.

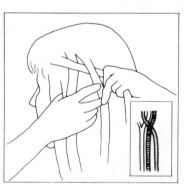

3   Gather a small section (about half as thick as one of the original strands) from the loose hair along your hairline next to the plait.

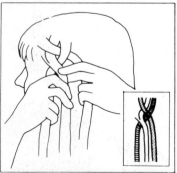

4   Add the gathered hair to the strand nearest your face and cross this increased strand over the centre, so that the two strands trade places.

Braided Face Frame

You can create several different looks with the Braided Face Frame by experimenting with the amount of hair you begin with and the thickness of the strands you add. Beginning with a very thin section

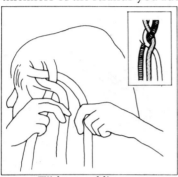

5 Without adding any new hair, cross the strand farthest from your face over the centre, so that these two strands trade places.

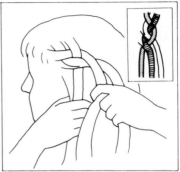

6 Gather a small section of the loose hair next to the braid. Add it to the strand nearest your face. Cross this increased strand over the centre.

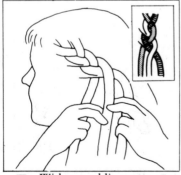

7 Without adding any new hair, cross the strand farthest from your face over the centre.

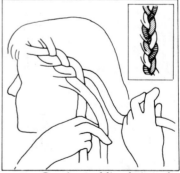

8 Continue adding hair to the strand nearest your face and crossing it over the centre, alternately crossing the far strand over the centre.

Braided Face Frame

of hair and adding very thin strands to it will result in a delicate accent braid; beginning with a thick section and adding thick strands to it will encircle your head with a bolder-looking braid.

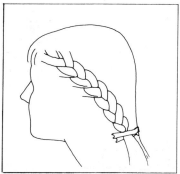

9 When the braid has nearly reached the nape of your neck, fasten it temporarily with a barrette, hair clip or hairpin.

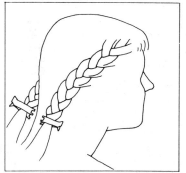

10 Repeat the same steps on the other side of your face, again beginning with the strand nearest your face. You'll have loose hair below the two braids.

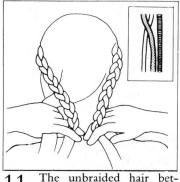

11 The unbraided hair between them becomes the centre strand of a new braid. Cross the left and then the right strand over the centre.

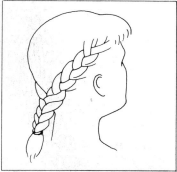

12 Remove the clips. Continue English braiding until the braid is complete. Fasten the end with a covered rubber band.

Hairline Twist with English Braid

The combination of a Hairline Twist with an English braid is one of the oldest and most classic of all braided styles. Slightly formal in appearance, it combines the standard English braid with a twisting technique to create an elegant look that's especially good for very long hair.

The Hairline Twist is a technique that, like braiding, is easy to

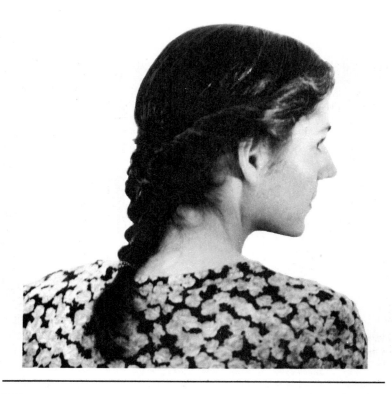

Hairline Twist with English Braid

learn. You begin by sectioning off a portion of hair on either side of your face. Then you wind the section back toward your nape while adding thin strands of hair gathered from the loose hair next to the

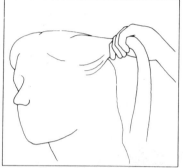

1 Beginning on your left side, section off a strand of hair from your hairline near your forehead. The strand should be about ½″ in diameter.

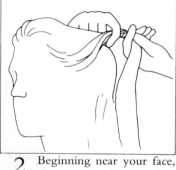

2 Beginning near your face, start to twist this strand up toward the top of your head. Hold it back, not down, as you twist.

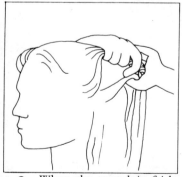

3 When the strand is fairly tight, gather a thin section from the loose hair near the twist and add it to the twisted strand.

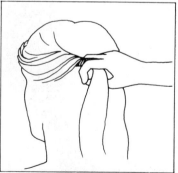

4 Continue adding thin sections to the twist and winding until the twisted hair nearly reaches your nape. Fasten it temporarily with a hair clip.

Hairline Twist with English Braid

hair being twisted. This technique gives you a "twist" of tightly wound hair that extends from your forehead to your nape, where it is temporarily fastened with hair clips. Once the twists are secured,

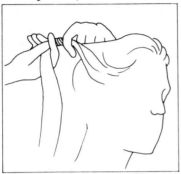

5 Section a strand of hair on your right side. Beginning near your face, twist it up towards the top of your head.

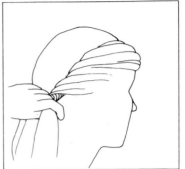

6 Continue winding and adding thin sections to the twist until the twisted hair nearly reaches the nape of your neck. Fasten it temporarily.

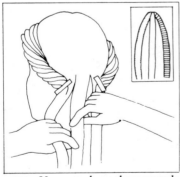

7 You now have three strands —two are partially twisted and fastened by hair clips, and one created by the loose, untwisted hair between those two strands.

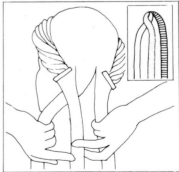

8 Cross the left strand over the centre, taking the centre strand to the left.

Hairline Twist with English Braid

you have loose hair beyond the hair clip on each twist, and loose hair in between them that hasn't been twisted at all. These three strands are simply English-braided.

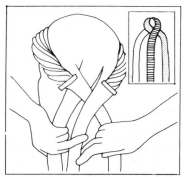

9 Cross the right strand over the centre, taking the centre strand to the right.

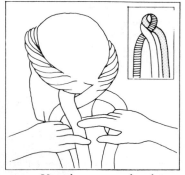

10 You have completed one plait. Remove the clips holding the two twisted strands.

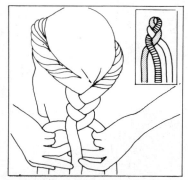

11 Continue crossing the left strand and then the right strand alternately over the centre until the braid is as long as you want it.

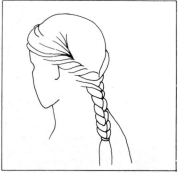

12 Fasten the end of the braid with a covered rubber band.

French Twist

French Twist

Although the French Twist is not technically a braid, it is included here because it closely resembles some of the more sophisticated braided styles. It is extremely easy to fashion; with a little practice, you'll be able to create this classic style in less than one minute.

Like braids, the French Twist is extremely practical. A properly fashioned French Twist will keep your hair elegantly in order all day.

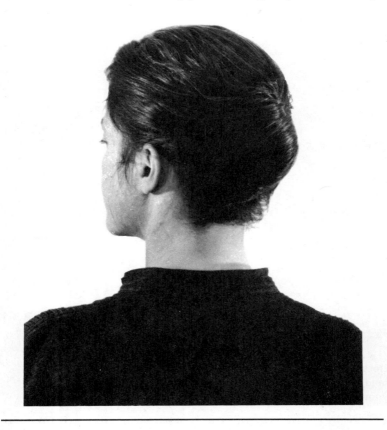

French Twist

A successful French Twist pulls all your hair smoothly away from your face to meet in a graceful, sloping roll at the left side of the back of your head.

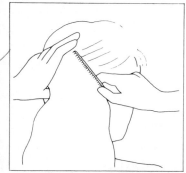

1   Comb your hair smoothly back from your forehead.

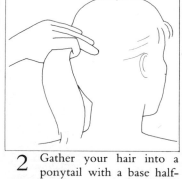

2   Gather your hair into a ponytail with a base half-way between your crown and nape and slightly to the left of centre. Don't anchor it.

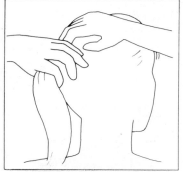

3   Twist the ponytail all the way around twice, in a clockwise direction. This will hold its base more closely against your head.

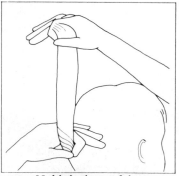

4   Hold the base of the pony-tail in your left hand. With your right, hold its end up, pointing toward the ceiling.

French Twist

Like braiding, creating a French Twist requires a combination of visualization and practice. When you look at a completed French Twist, it is difficult to imagine how it was fashioned. The step-by-

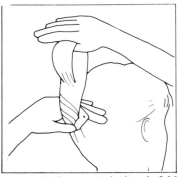

5 With your right hand, fold the end of the ponytail (about the top third) down toward your nape.

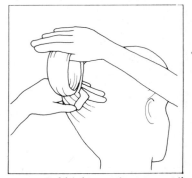

6 Fold the entire ponytail down under itself, toward your nape, so that it is less than half as long as it was.

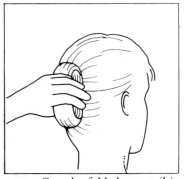

7 Cup the folded ponytail in your left hand. There should be a slight hollow between the ponytail and your scalp.

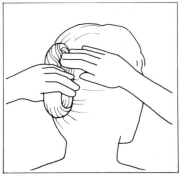

8 With your right hand, begin to gently push the upper right-hand portion of the folded ponytail down into the hollow.

French Twist

step illustrations below, however, will show you how easy it is. Imagine yourself carrying out each of the steps on your own hair before you begin.

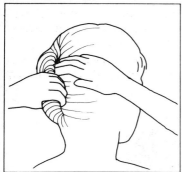

9 Continue pushing the hair underneath your left hand into the hollow, so that the folded ponytail is slowly rolling inside the hollow.

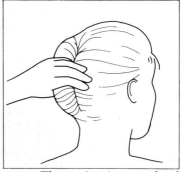

10 The twist is completed when you can't push any additional hair into the hollow, and the folded ponytail has become a tight roll.

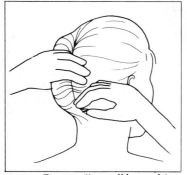

11 Create a "seam" by tucking in bobby pins along the line formed where the right hand edge of the roll meets your scalp, starting at the bottom.

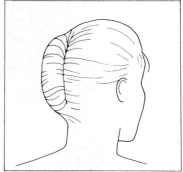

12 Place bobby pins all along the "seam," up to the top of the roll, concealing them just under the roll.

Underbraid

Underbraid

The glamorous Underbraid appears elaborate and intricate, but it is actually just as easy to fashion as a French braid. It combines French and Dutch braiding techniques to create a stunning braid that stands out from your head, surrounded by gracefully draped hair.

The Underbraid is, in fact, the opposite of a French braid. Instead of hiding the braided ponytail underneath the gathers of hair, the

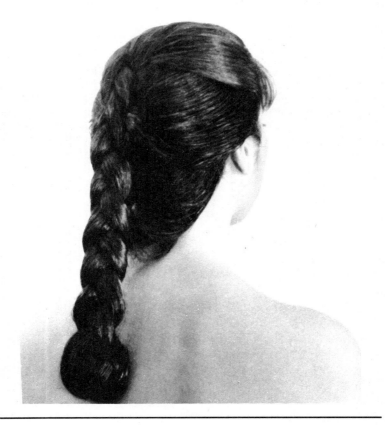

Underbraid

Underbraid uses the gathered hair as a base underneath the braid, causing it to stand out.

Because the Underbraid is created using motions that may seem

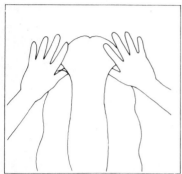

1 Place your thumbs above and behind your ears. Draw your thumbs slightly back and upward, gathering the hair that meets at your crown in a ponytail.

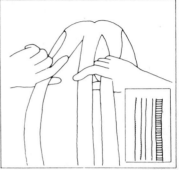

2 Divide the ponytail into three approximately equal strands and position your fingers to begin braiding.

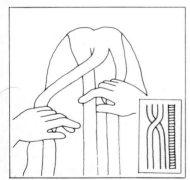

3 Cross the left strand under the centre, taking the centre strand to the left.

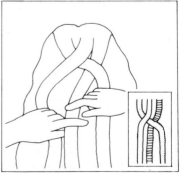

4 Cross the right strand under the centre, taking the centre strand to the right.

Underbraid

unfamiliar at first, it's important that you use the hand positions and movements that feel most comfortable to you. These illustrations show a braider using her own individual technique. As long as you

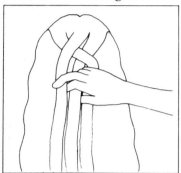

5 Hold the plait in your right hand, separating the three loose strands below it with your fingers.

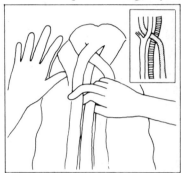

6 Place your left thumb above and slightly behind your ear. Draw a strand half as thick as one of the original strands toward the ponytail.

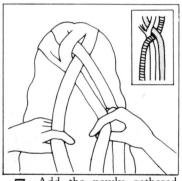

7 Add the newly gathered hair to the left strand. Cross the increased left strand under the centre, taking the centre strand to the left.

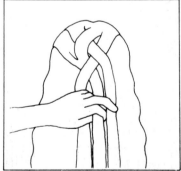

8 Hold the plait in your left hand, separating the three loose strands below it with your fingers.

Underbraid

fashion one Dutch plait and then begin gathering hair and crossing the increased strands **under** the centre, it really doesn't matter how you do it.

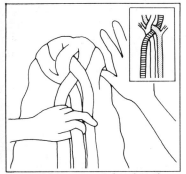

9 Use your right thumb to draw a strand about half as thick as one of the original strands toward the ponytail.

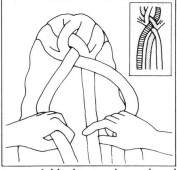

10 Add the newly gathered hair to the right strand. Cross the increased right strand under the centre, taking the centre strand to the right.

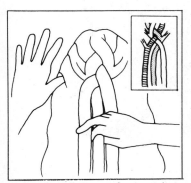

11 Continue gathering hair from the left and right and adding to the strands just before you cross them under the centre.

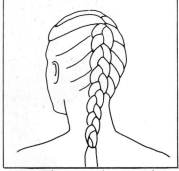

12 When you have no loose hair left to gather, Dutch-braid the strands that are left. Fasten the end with a covered rubber band.

The Cameo

The Cameo

This classic style, often pictured on cameo jewellery, is an appealingly formal look that requires fairly long hair and a bit of patience.

A simple chignon, or bun, is the basis of the Cameo. If you don't have experience in creating a chignon, don't worry. Our illustrations show a braider using a chignon foundation, a doughnut-shaped nylon mesh object available at most hairdresseres and department stores.

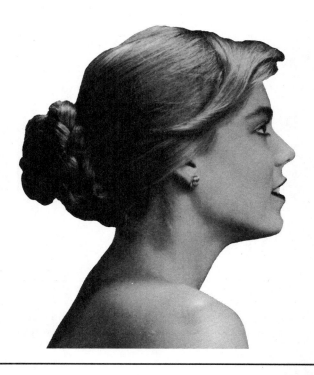

The Cameo

You'll gather your hair into a ponytail, draw the ponytail through the hole in the foundation, then spread the strands over the rounded

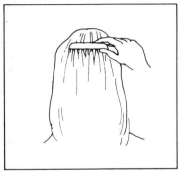

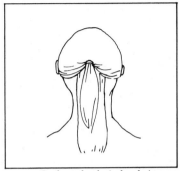

1 Comb your hair straight back from your forehead to eliminate the parting.

2 Gather the hair back into a ponytail with its base half-way between crown and nape and anchor it with a covered rubber band. Leave a two-inch-wide section of loose hair hanging below it.

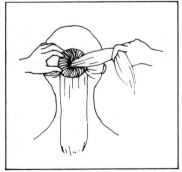

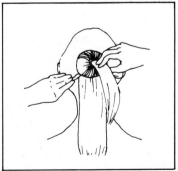

3 Pull the ponytail through the centre of the foundation, bringing the foundation up against your head.

4 Take a small section of hair and gently smooth it over the edge of the foundation. Use a hairpin to fasten it underneath.

The Cameo

edges of the foundation, pinning them invisibly underneath it to create a perfect chignon. You'll complete the look by English-

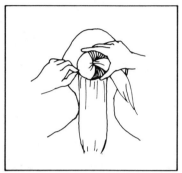

5   Take another small section next to the first one and gently smooth it over the edge of the foundation, using a hairpin to fasten it underneath.

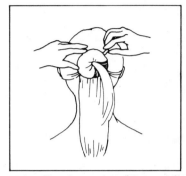

6   Continue smoothing small sections of hair over the edge of the foundation, carefully concealing their ends underneath and fastening them with hairpins.

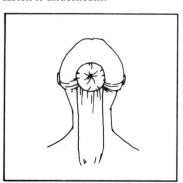

7   When the ponytail has been tucked around the foundation, you should have a neat chignon with a section of loose hair hanging below it.

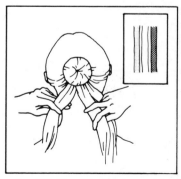

8   Divide the loose section into three approximately equal strands and position your fingers to begin braiding.

The Cameo

braiding the loose section of hair at your nape and wrapping it around the chignon.

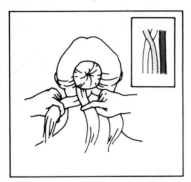

9 Cross the left strand over the centre, taking the centre strand to the left, so that the two strands trade places.

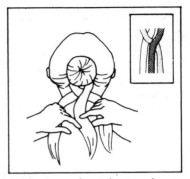

10 Cross the right strand over the centre, taking the centre strand to the right, so that these two strands trade places.

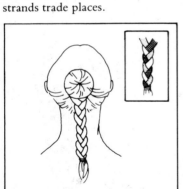

11 Continue English-braiding. When you reach the bottom of the strands, fasten them with a covered rubber band.

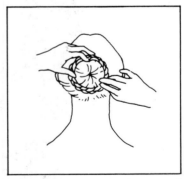

12 Bring the braid up and around the chignon, encircling its base. Tuck the end of the braid under the bottom of the chignon and secure it firmly in place with hairpins.

Ribbon Braid

Ribbon Braid

This easy-to-make braid is surprisingly versatile and festive. The look varies with the colour of the accent you choose to weave in with the English braids.

Make sure that the ribbon or yarn you're weaving in with the braids is at least two or three inches longer than your hair, so there'll be some left over to conceal the rubber band that fastens the braid. Don't worry if the ribbon is too long—you can always trim the ends when you've finished braiding.

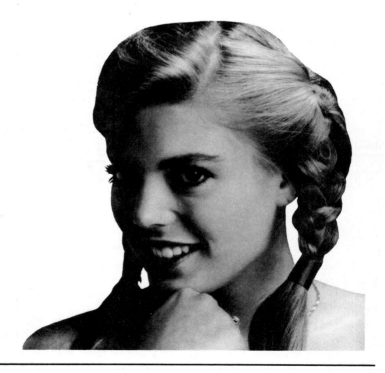

Ribbon Braid

You needn't anchor the ribbon in place. When the braid is fashioned properly, it's very taut and the tension between the strands keeps the ribbon secure.

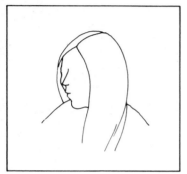

1 Part your hair from the centre of your forehead to the nape. The parting must be very straight.

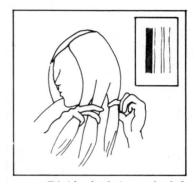

2 Divide the hair on the left side of the parting into three approximately equal strands.

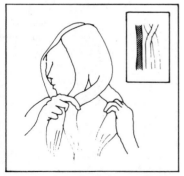

3 Cross the left strand over the centre, taking the centre strand to the left, so that the two strands trade places.

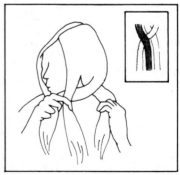

4 Cross the right strand over the centre, taking the centre strand to the right, so that these two strands trade places.

Ribbon Braid

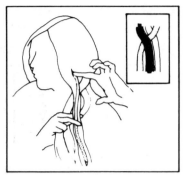

5   Hold all three strands in one hand. With the other, carefully lay the ribbon along the centre strand, concealing its end underneath a strand of the plait.

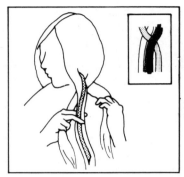

6   The ribbon is now a part of the strand that's currently in the centre.

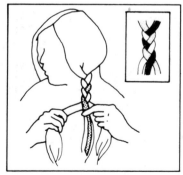

7   Continue regular English-braiding, crossing the left and then the right strands over the centre. The ribbon stays with its original strand.

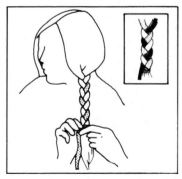

8   When you reach the bottom of the strands, fasten the ends with a covered rubber band. Let the ribbon hang below the strands.

Ribbon Braid

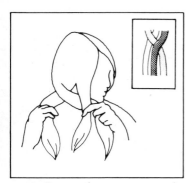

9 Repeat the sequence on the right side. Cross the left and then the right strand over the centre.

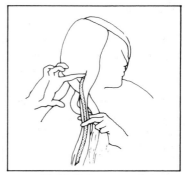

10 Hold all three strands in one hand. With the other, carefully lay the ribbon along the centre strand, concealing its end underneath a strand of the plait.

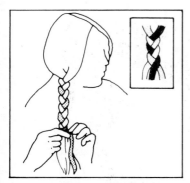

11 Continue English-braiding, keeping the ribbon with its original strand. Fasten the end of the braid with a covered rubber band.

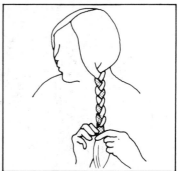

12 Wrap the loose ends of the ribbons around the covered rubber bands. You can secure the ends by tucking them under the wrapped ribbon and into the covered rubber band, or by firmly pressing invisible cellophane tape against the end of the ribbon.

The Tiara

The Tiara

Practically everybody has, at one time or another, fashioned braided pigtails—one English braid on either side of the head. They're easy to make and perfect for keeping your hair in order and out of your way.

Mothers of little girls especially appreciate the practical and durable characteristics of this look. But, like most braids, these braided pigtails can be more than practical. They can easily be turned into a stylish look simply by using them to encircle the head in a Tiara.

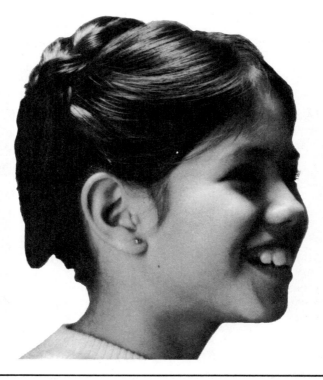

The Tiara

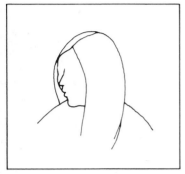

1 Part your hair from the centre of your forehead to the nape. The parting must be very straight.

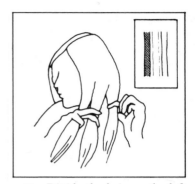

2 Divide the hair on the left side of the part into three approximately equal strands. You can hold the strands taut, so that the braid begins high on your hair, or loosely, so that the braid begins below the ear.

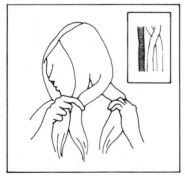

3 Cross the left strand over the centre, taking the centre strand to the left, so that the two strands trade places.

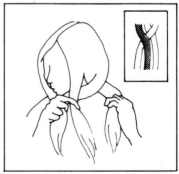

4 Cross the right strand over the centre, taking the centre strand to the right, so that these two strands trade places.

The Tiara

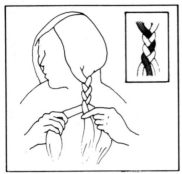

5 Continue English-braiding, crossing the left and then the right strands over the centre.

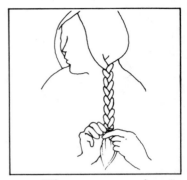

6 When you reach the bottom of the strands, fasten the ends with a covered rubber band.

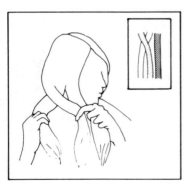

7 Repeat the sequence on the right side. Cross the left strand over the centre, taking the centre strand to the left, so that the two strands trade places.

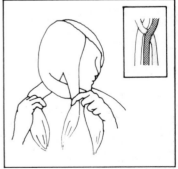

8 Cross the right strand over the centre, taking the centre strand to the right, so that these two strands trade places.

The Tiara

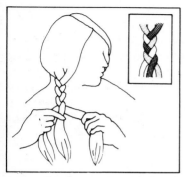

9 Continue English-braiding, crossing the left and then the right strand over the centre.

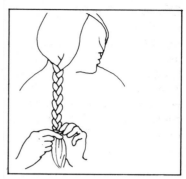

10 When you reach the bottom of the strands, fasten the ends with a covered rubber band.

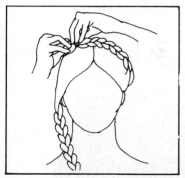

11 Bring the left braid up and lay it flat against your head with its end pointing toward your right ear. Secure it to the scalp with hairpins.

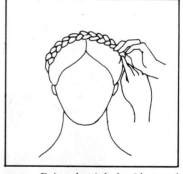

12 Bring the right braid up and lay it flat against your head with its end pointing toward your left ear. Conceal the ends of both braids beneath the plaits and fasten the second braid to your scalp with hairpins.

Duchess Braid

Duchess Braid

The Duchess braid, a single braid that frames the face, is fashioned using a variation of the French-braiding technique. Ideal for keeping bangs that are growing out neatly away from your face, the Duchess is unusual in that it requires you to begin the braid on one side of your face, gradually braid up toward the top of your head, and then continue down along the other side of your face. Gathering hair from behind the braid and adding it to the strands as you work keeps

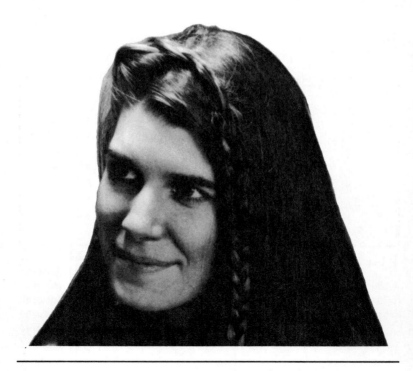

Duchess Braid

the finished Duchess braid anchored firmly to the loose hair behind it.

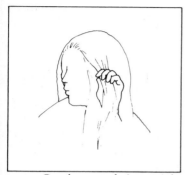

1 Comb your hair straight back from your forehead to eliminate the parting, and gather a one-inch-thick section of hair from your hairline just above the temple.

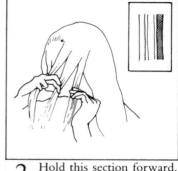

2 Hold this section forward, with its end extending past your face, and divide it into three approximately equal strands.

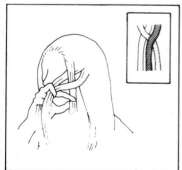

3 Fashion one English plait by crossing the left and the right strand over the centre, then hold the plait and loose strands below it with one hand.

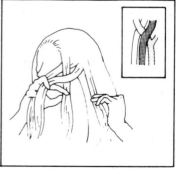

4 Gather a section of hair about as thick as one of the strands from the loose hair directly behind the braid.

Duchess Braid

Although the illustrations show a braider beginning the braid with a one-inch-thick section of hair, you can create a variety of

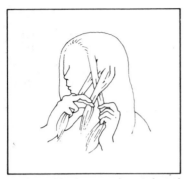

5   Add the newly gathered hair to the strand farthest from your face, then cross this increased strand over the centre.

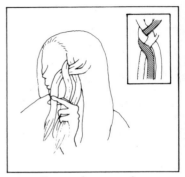

6   Cross the strand nearest your face over the centre without gathering any hair, then hold the plaits and loose hair below them in one hand.

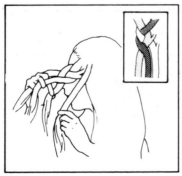

7   Lift the braid slightly toward the top of your head and gather another thin section from the loose hair directly behind it.

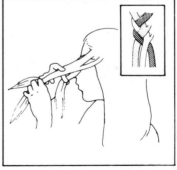

8   Add the hair to the strand farthest from your face and cross this increased section over the centre strand.

Duchess Braid

looks with the Duchess braid simply by beginning with different-sized sections of hair.

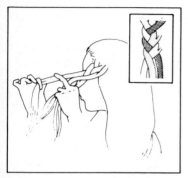

9 Cross the section nearest your face over the centre without adding any hair.

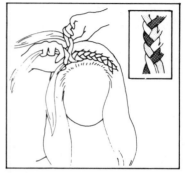

10 Repeat steps 7 through 9, working the braid up past the top of your head and down the other side of your face.

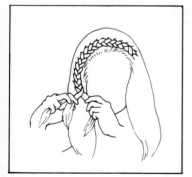

11 When the base of the braid is even with the bottom of your ear, stop gathering hair.

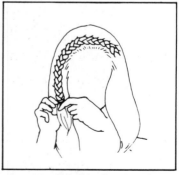

12 English-braid the loose strands and fasten the end with a covered rubber band.

Princess Braid

This look was made famous by Princess Leia in the movie *Star Wars*. In fact, this arrangement of English braids dates back to the fourteenth century, when nearly all women had very long hair and frequently wore braids to keep their hair arranged neatly.

The Princess braid looks good on girls and women of all ages. It works on hair that's slightly above shoulder length or longer. If your hair is at the shorter end of this range, the braided loops you fashion at the sides of your head will be fairly compact. If your hair is very

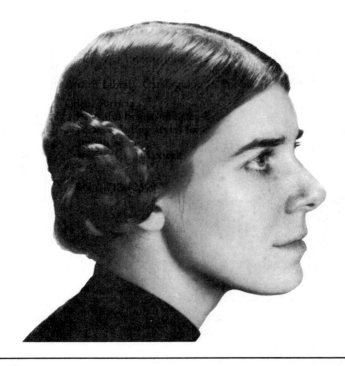

Princess Braid

long, you can create longer loops or wrap the braids into two or more loops. The choice is yours.

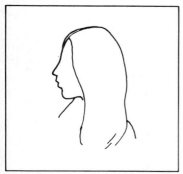

1 Part your hair from the centre of your forehead to the nape. The parting must be very straight.

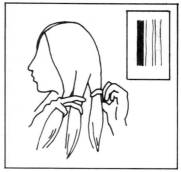

2 Divide the hair on the left side of the part into three approximately equal strands.

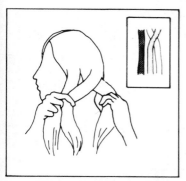

3 Cross the left strand over the centre, taking the centre strand to the left, so that the two strands trade places.

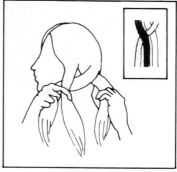

4 Cross the right strand over the centre, taking the centre strand to the right, so that these two strands trade places.

Princess Braid

Our illustrations show a braider beginning on the left side, but you can begin on either side.

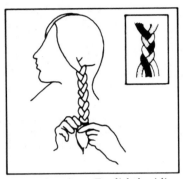

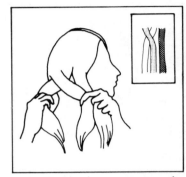

5 Continue English-braiding until you reach the bottom of the stands, then fasten the end with a covered rubber band.

6 Repeat the sequence on the right side. Cross the left strand over the centre, taking the centre strand to the left.

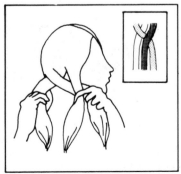

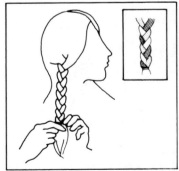

7 Cross the right strand over the centre, taking the centre strand to the right, so that the two strands trade places.

8 Continue English-braiding until you reach the bottom of the strands, then fasten the end with a covered rubber band.

Princess Braid

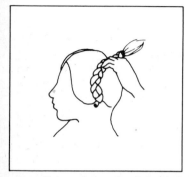

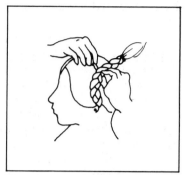

9 Bring the end of the left braid up so that the back of the braid is parallel to your face and curved slightly toward the back of your head. The portion of the braid near the top of your ear will be the midpoint.

10 Use a hairpin to fasten the midpoint of the braid to the hair near the top of your ear.

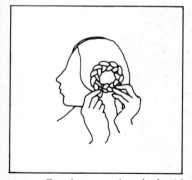

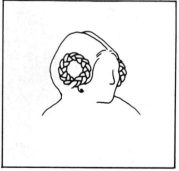

11 Continue curving the braid down around the back of your ear, concealing the braid's end under its base and securing it with a hairpin.

12 Use several hairpins to secure the loop firmly to the hair around it, then repeat on the other side.

Simplified Cornrows

Simplified Cornrows

Cornrows are among the most famous of all the braided styles. Like braids themselves, they come in all shapes, sizes, and levels of complexity. Although cornrows were popularized by Bo Derek in the 1979 film *10*, the look is actually a traditional African style that dates at least as far back as the sixteenth century.

A truly expert cornrower can sculpt hair into swirling or symmetrical patterns against the scalp, but even the novice braider can create an intricate cornrow look by fashioning a series of tiny Dutch braids. You can leave the tiny braids hanging loose, but we show them gathered into elaborate pigtails for a more "finished"

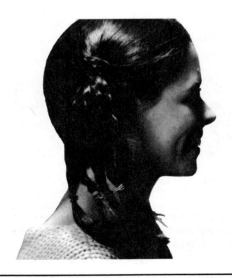

Simplified Cornrows

look. You can also draw the Dutch braids into a thick braided ponytail.

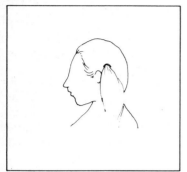

1 Part your hair from the centre of your forehead to the nape. The parting must be very straight. Gather the hair on each side into a ponytail, with its base anchored firmly against the side of your head.

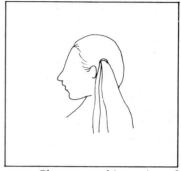

2 Choose one thin section of hair to braid first. (Decide how many braids you want to create before choosing the width of this section.)

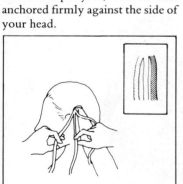

3 Divide the section into three approximately even strands and position your fingers to begin braiding.

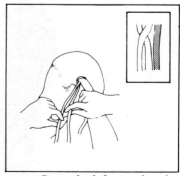

4 Cross the left strand under the centre strand, pulling them taut, so that the left strand and the centre strand trade places.

Simplified Cornrows

Simplified cornrows can be fashioned from all hair types—straight or curly, thin or coarse. The number of braids you fashion

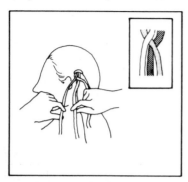

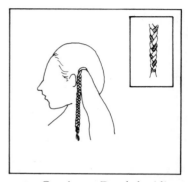

5 Cross the right strand under the centre strand, pulling them taut, so that the right strand and the centre strand trade places.

6 Continue Dutch-braiding until you reach the bottom of the strands, then fasten the end with a covered rubber band.

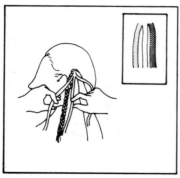

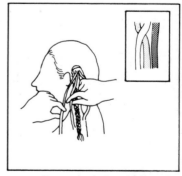

7 Take another section and divide it into three approximately equal strands. Position your fingers to begin braiding.

8 Cross the left strand under the centre strand, pulling them taut, so that the left strand and the centre strand trade places.

Simplified Cornrows

depends on the thickness of your hair and the time you're willing to spend working.

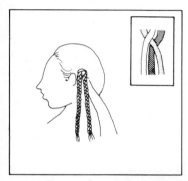

9 Cross the right strand under the centre strand, pulling them taut, so that the right strand and the centre strand trade places. Repeat steps 6 through 9 until there is no loose hair left.

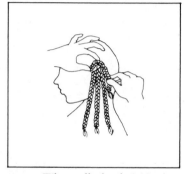

10 When all the hair in one ponytail has been braided, select one braid and wrap it around the covered rubber band that's holding the braids together.

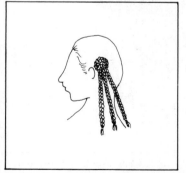

11 Conceal the end of the wrapper braid underneath the covered rubber band.

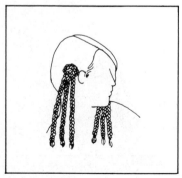

12 Repeat on the other side.

Parisian Braid

Parisian Braid

This pretty and practical accent braid will ornament your hair while keeping it drawn neatly back from your face.

You can create the Parisian braid in a variety of sizes. Beginning with a fairly thick section of hair will give you a wide, sturdy-looking braid; beginning with a thin section will yield a delicate, slightly wispy-looking braid. Try it both ways and see which one suits you best.

While using the elegant French braid to create this style gives your hair a particularly dressy look, English or Dutch braids work just as well.

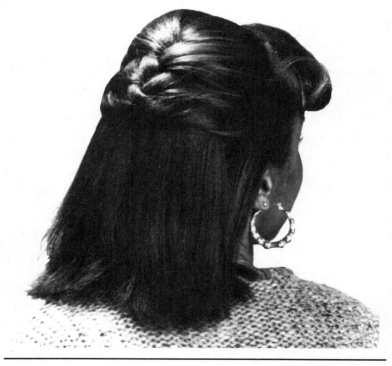

Parisian Braid

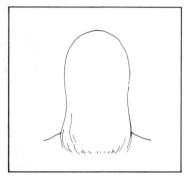

1 Comb your hair straight back from your forehead to eliminate the parting.

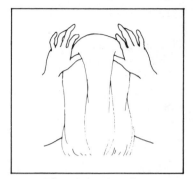

2 Place your thumbs at your hairline, even with your eyes. Draw them back and slightly upward toward your crown, gathering hair as they move.

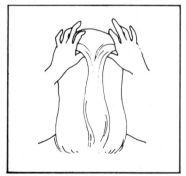

3 Your thumbs should meet at your crown, creating a thin ponytail skimmed from the top layer of hair. Don't anchor it.

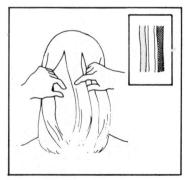

4 Divide this thin ponytail into three approximately equal strands and position your fingers to begin braiding.

Parisian Braid

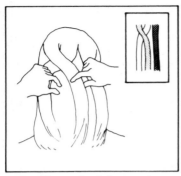

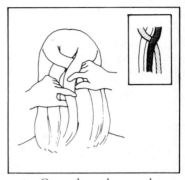

5 Cross the left strand over the centre, taking the centre strand to the left.

6 Cross the right strand over the centre, taking the centre strand to the right.

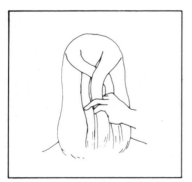

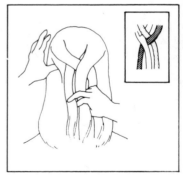

7 Hold the plait in your right hand, its loose strands separated by your fingers.

8 Use your left thumb to gather a very thin strand from the loose hair at the left of the braid. Add it to the left strand and cross this increased strand over the centre, taking the centre strand to the left.

Parisian Braid

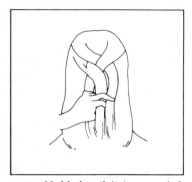

9 Hold the plait in your left hand, its loose strands separated by your fingers.

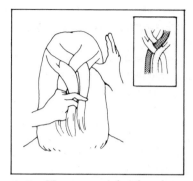

10 Use your right thumb to gather a very thin strand from the loose hair at the right of the braid. Add it to the right strand and cross this increased strand over the centre, taking the centre strand to the right.

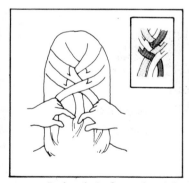

11 Gather hair from the right and left and add it to the strands just before crossing them over the centre until the strands are braided halfway down.

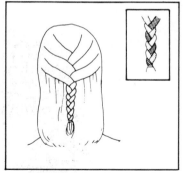

12 English-braid the loose strands until the braid is as long as you want it, then fasten the end with a covered rubber band. You can tuck the hanging portion of the braid up underneath the French plaits and secure it with hairpins.

Gainsborough Braid

Gainsborough Braid

This nineteenth-century English braid arrangement was considered a suitable daytime style for young women. In the more casual twentieth century, the Gainsborough braid is ideal for special occasions.

Because the style requires that you create and arrange four separate braids, it's best to try it on a friend first. You'll see how simple it really is, and it will be much easier when you try it on yourself.

If you want to try it on your own hair first, remember to visualize each step as you work. As you complete each braid, clip it out of your way so you can fashion the others without becoming confused.

The instructions are written so you can follow them when you're braiding your own hair, and the illustrations show a braider using the instructions on someone else's hair.

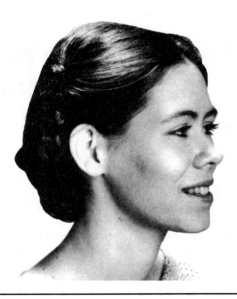

Gainsborough Braid

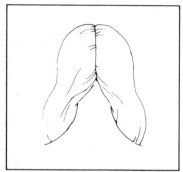

1 Part your hair from the centre of your forehead to the nape. The parting must be very straight.

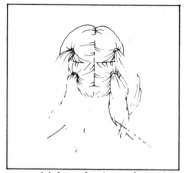

2 Make a horizontal parting running from ear to ear, so that your hair is divided into four equal sections. Pull each section into a ponytail anchored with a covered rubber band to keep them separate.

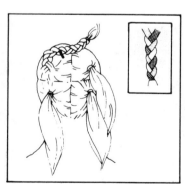

3 Remove the band from the front left ponytail and English-braid only this section of hair, fastening the end of the braid with the covered rubber band. Clip the finished braid out of your way.

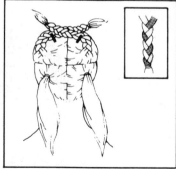

4 Remove the band from the front right ponytail and English-braid only this section of hair, fastening the end of the braid with the covered rubber band. Clip the finished braid out of your way.

Gainsborough Braid

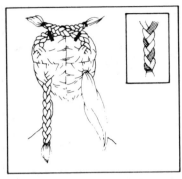

5 Remove the band from the back left ponytail and English-braid this section of hair, fastening the end of the braid with the covered rubber band.

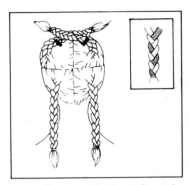

6 Remove the band from the back right ponytail and English-braid this section of hair, fastening the end of the braid with the covered rubber band.

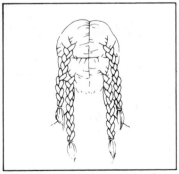

7 Unclip the two front braids, letting all four hang down the back of your head.

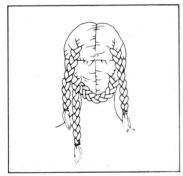

8 Bring the back right braid across the nape of your neck, tucking its end under the base of the back left braid. Fasten the end securely to the left braid's base with a hairpin.

Gainsborough Braid

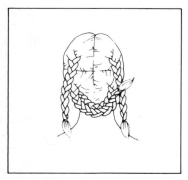

9 Bring the back left braid across the nape of your neck, crossing it over the right braid.

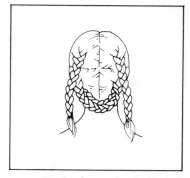

10 Tuck the end of the left braid under the base of the right and fasten it with a hairpin.

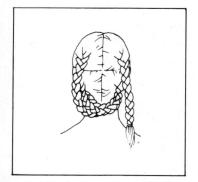

11 Tuck the end of the right front braid underneath the braids at your nape and pin it in place.

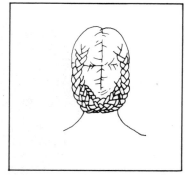

12 Tuck the end of the left front braid underneath the braids at your nape and pin it in place.

Evensong

Evensong

This stunning style results from combining French and Dutch braiding techniques to create two braids that stand out from your head.

In the Evensong style, you'll begin by fashioning two Dutch braids, but you'll also use the French-braiding technique of gathering and adding hair to strands. Because you'll be crossing these increased strands under, rather than over, the centre strand of each braid, the finished braid will be elevated from your scalp, with each detail of the braid clearly visible.

The hand motions necessary for creating a Dutch braid while gathering hair into the strands may feel a little awkward, so try it on a friend first so you can see how it works. Remember, all you really have to do is fashion two Dutch braids, one at a time, while adding loose hair to the left and right strands.

The instructions are written so you can follow them when you're braiding your own hair, and the illustrations show a braider using the instructions on someone else's hair.

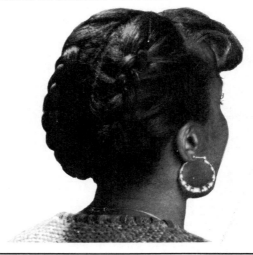

Evensong

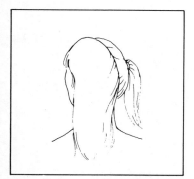

1 Part your hair from the centre of your forehead to the nape. The parting must be very straight. Gather the hair on one side into a ponytail to keep it out of your way.

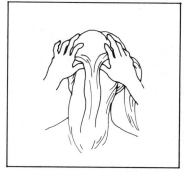

2 On the other side, place one thumb against your temple and the other parallel to it at your parting. Draw your thumbs toward each other and slightly upward, gathering the top layer of loose hair into a thin ponytail that is the basis of the first Dutch braid.

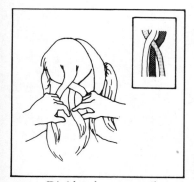

3 Divide the ponytail into three strands and fashion one Dutch plait by crossing the left and then the right strand under the centre strand.

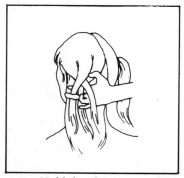

4 Hold the plait in your right hand, separating the loose strands below it with your fingers.

Evensong

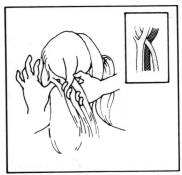

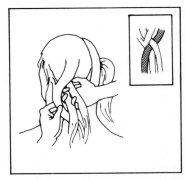

5 Place your left thumb near your face, slightly below the plait. Draw a strand half as thick as one of the original strands toward the plait and add it to the left strand.

6 Cross the increased strand under the centre strand, taking the centre strand to the left.

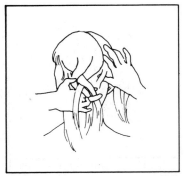

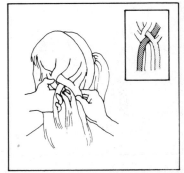

7 Hold the plait in your left hand, separating the loose strands below it with your fingers. Place your right thumb at the parting, slightly below the plait.

8 Draw a strand half as thick as one of the original strands toward the plait and add it to the right strand.

Evensong

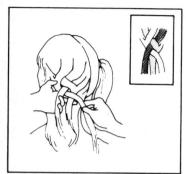

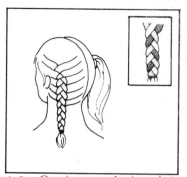

9   Cross this increased strand under the centre strand, taking the centre strand to the right.

10   Continue gathering hair from the left and right and adding it to the strands just before you cross them under the centre. When there is no more hair left to gather, Dutch-braid the strands and fasten the end with a covered rubber band.

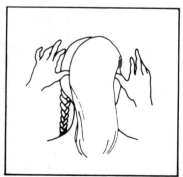

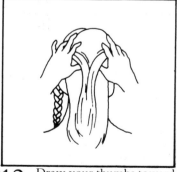

11   Unfasten the ponytail on the other side and place one thumb against your temple and the other parallel to it at your parting.

12   Draw your thumbs toward each other and slightly upward, gathering the top layer of loose hair into a thin ponytail, which is the basis of the second Dutch braid.

Evensong

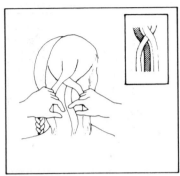

13 Divide the ponytail into three strands and fashion one Dutch plait by crossing the left and then the right strand under the centre strand.

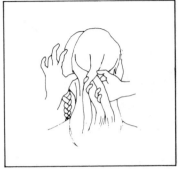

14 Hold the plait in your right hand, separating the loose strands below it with your fingers. Place your left thumb at the parting, slightly below the plait.

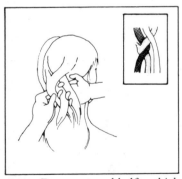

15 Draw a strand half as thick as one of the original strands toward the plait. Add this newly gathered hair to the left strand and cross this increased strand under the centre strand, taking the centre strand to the left.

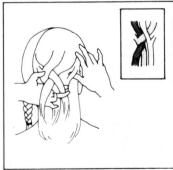

16 Hold the plait in your left hand, separating the loose strand below it with your fingers. Place your right thumb near your face, slightly below the plait. Draw a strand half as thick as one of the original strands toward the plait and add it to the right strand.

Evensong

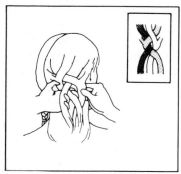

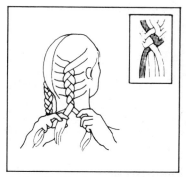

17 Cross this increased strand under the centre strand, taking the centre strand to the right.

18 Continue gathering hair from the left and right and adding it to the strands just before you cross them under the centre.

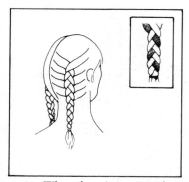

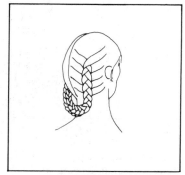

19 When there is no more hair left to gather, Dutch-braid the strands and fasten the end with a covered rubber band.

20 Cross the braids at your nape, fastening each end underneath the opposite braid with a hairpin.

Josephine's Braids

Josephine's Braids

This sophisticated look is created by partially fashioning one French and one combination French-Dutch braid, one above the other, then combining the loose strands of both braids, English-braiding them together, and coiling them into a chignon.

It's important to position each braid. Remember that you want the finished chignon to be about midway between your crown and nape, so the top braid should begin high up on your head, just below the crown.

The instructions are written so you can follow them when you're braiding your own hair, and the illustrations show a braider using the instructions on someone else's hair.

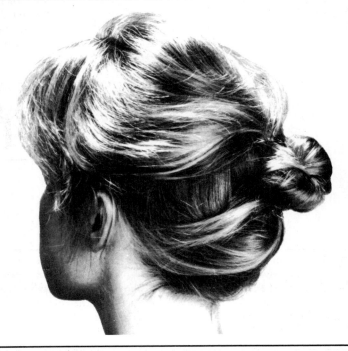

Josephine's Braids

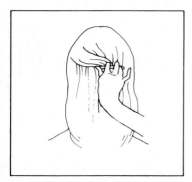

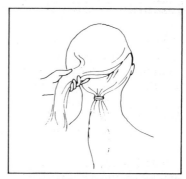

1 Comb your hair straight back from your forehead and make a horizontal parting running from ear to ear, dividing your hair into two equal sections.

2 You'll work with the top section first, so gather the bottom section into a ponytail and fasten it with a covered rubber band to keep it out of your way.

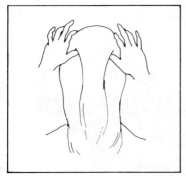

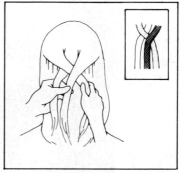

3 Place your thumbs at your hairline, even with your eyes, and draw them up to your crown to create a thin ponytail skimmed from the top layer of hair.

4 Divide this hair into three nearly equal strands and fashion one English plait by taking the left and then the right strand over the centre.

Josephine's Braids

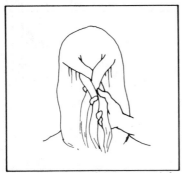

5   Hold the plait in your right hand, separating the loose strands below it with your fingers.

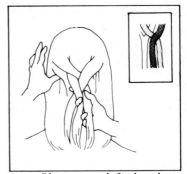

6   Place your left thumb at your hairline, even with the top of your eyebrow. Use it to gather a strand half as thick as one of the original strands from the loose hair and add it to the left strand.

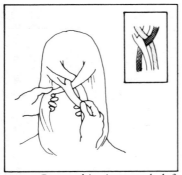

7   Cross this increased left strand over the centre, pulling it taut, so that the centre strand and the left strand trade places.

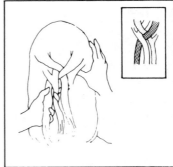

8   Place your right thumb at your hairline, even with the top of your eyebrow. Use it to gather a strand half as thick as one of the original strands from the loose hair and add it to the right strand.

Josephine's Braids

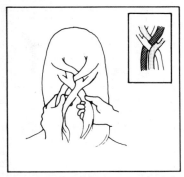

9 Cross this increased right strand over the centre, pulling it taut. The centre strand and the right strand trade places.

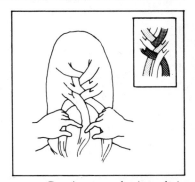

10 Continue gathering hair from the left and right and adding it to the strands just before you cross them over the centre.

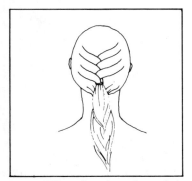

11 When there is no loose hair left to gather, fasten the unbraided strands tightly together with a covered rubber band just below the plaits.

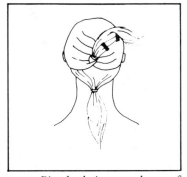

12 Pin the hair up and out of your way. You will use a combination of French and Dutch braiding techniques on the bottom section of hair.

Josephine's Braids

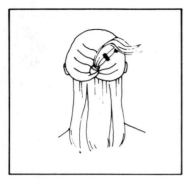

13 Unfasten the bottom pony-tail dividing it into three sections. The centre section should be about twice as thick as the two other sections.

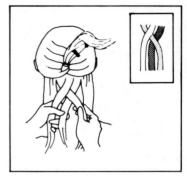

14 Divide the centre section into three equal strands and fashion one Dutch plait, crossing the left and then the right strand under the centre.

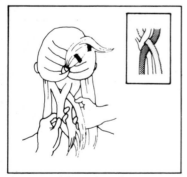

15 Holding the plait in your right hand, gather about a third of the hair from the left section, adding it to the left strand of the centre section. Cross this increased left strand under the centre strand, taking the centre strand to the left.

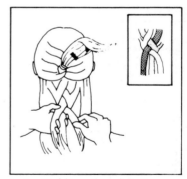

16 Holding the plait in your left hand, gather about a third of the hair from the right section, adding it to the right strand of the centre section. Cross this increased right strand under the centre strand, taking the centre strand to the right.

Josephine's Braids

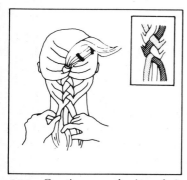

17 Continue gathering hair from the left and right sections and adding it to the left and right strands of the centre section before crossing them under the centre.

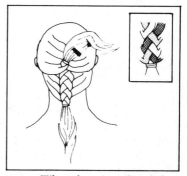

18 When there is no hair left to gather from the side sections, fasten the unbraided strands tightly together with a covered rubber band placed just below the Dutch plaits.

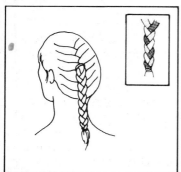

19 Bring the loose hair from the French and Dutch braids together in a ponytail fastened with a covered rubber band. English-braid the ponytail.

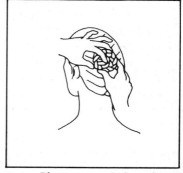

20 Place your index finger against your head, touching the base of the braid, and coil the braid around it. Use hairpins to secure the coil tightly to your scalp, concealing the end of the English braid underneath the coil.

Dress Up Your Braids

Our photographs and illustrations have shown you how to create braids and braided styles; now it's up to you to experiment and add your own finishing touches. Each style we've shown can be adapted and combined with others, once you've mastered the techniques. For example, you can easily fashion two Dutch braids, one on either side of your head, by modifying the instructions given for the single Dutch braid. And, using the basic instructions, you can fashion two French braids at the back of your head or a single English braid on the side.

If you want an altogether new look, now you can add-a-braid! It is possible to buy a braid as long as 24" made from synthetic fibre to match any hair colour. Mix and match it with your natural braids, tie it around your head, twist it into a bun, let it dangle like a pigtail. Experiment, and remember that the placement of braids is up to you.

You can also highlight your favourite braided looks with accessories. Barrettes and hair clips come in a range of colours, shapes and sizes, and even ornamented wire hairpins are widely available. They all decorate the hair they're holding. For an elegant look, try adding a delicate comb to an Invisible French braid, or pierce a braided Chignon with exotic-looking chopsticks. Also try accessories that aren't just for hair. Weave a thin strand of beads in with a Braided Face Frame, or fasten the end of an English or Dutch braid with brightly coloured ribbons or yarn. The choices are yours.